Meningococcal Disease:

My Encounter with the Infection and Essential Information You Must Know

Written by

Dr. Judy Medina

Copyright © by Dr. Judy Medina 2023. All rights reserved.

Table of Contents

My Encounter with the Infection

A scary and sometimes fatal condition, meningococcal disease can affect anyone, at any stage of life, without prior notice.

My own journey through this terrifying experience proved to be a tale of survival, tenacity, and newly discovered gratitude for life. I had no idea that after serving, I would end up in the hospital when I was chosen to participate in a medical mission for freshly enlisted soldiers in a military base.

Fever, headache, and excessive weariness were the first symptoms I noticed, which I originally brushed off as the flu. I had no idea that these seemingly unremarkable indications were actually the early indications of a fatal bacterial infection. I was brought to the hospital as my condition began to decline over the course of the following days. The bleak prognosis indicated that I had meningococcal illness, an infection caused by bacteria that damages the membranes protecting the brain and spinal cord.

The following few days were a haze of medical treatments from bloodstream infection and anxiety. I was given critical treatment, where a group of committed medical specialists worked nonstop to preserve my life. I was in serious danger of developing a severe impairment or maybe passing away because the sickness had advanced so quickly. Even though the deck was stacked against me, I was willing to fight.

My path to rehabilitation wasn't without its difficulties. I went through a long and difficult rehabilitation process, as well as agony. The path was paved with obstacles, but I took courage from my loved ones' steadfast support. Their support and affection helped me get through each challenge, and they became my lifeline.

Meningococcal illness is no longer practically a death sentence thanks to advances regarding early diagnosis, treatment with antibiotics, and vaccination. My experience made clear how crucial it is to spread knowledge about the illness and promote immunization in order to stop its effects.

I am a meningococcal illness survivor today. I have a newfound zest for life and a profound appreciation for every moment as a result of this profoundly transformative event. In order to encourage others to find their own inner resilience and not to overlook their health for granted, I'm dedicated to sharing my story.

I hope that my experience can serve as a source of inspiration for those going through similar hardships, showing them that they can survive while understanding that each day is a priceless gift to be treasured.

An Overview of the Disease

Any health condition brought on by the Neisseria Meningitidis bacterium is referred to as meningococcal disease. Meningitis and bloodstream infections are among the serious, frequently fatal disorders that fall under this category. It results in inflammation of the membranes that surround spinal cord and the brain.

Without timely treatment, meningococcal meningitis could prove deadly or extremely harmful. The causative germs are spread through aerosols, and by coming into close interaction with someone who has been infected. Activities like coughing, kissing, or sneezing might cause this. In overcrowded or close-contact environments like military camps, dorms, and homes, it occurs more frequently.

Meningococcal disease can cause a number of issues, such as damage to the brain, seizures, hearing loss, difficulty seeing, amputation of limbs, and even death, if it is not treated in a timely manner. Some of these issues may become chronic and long-term affecting someone's well-being and standard of life.

Bacterial Strains That Cause Meningococcal Infection

The most frequent strain of bacteria responsible for bacterial meningitis is Streptococcus pneumoniae. This kind of bacteria is the most frequent cause of bacterial meningitis in children and adults.

Below are the strains of bacteria that can trigger an infection;

Meningitis caused by Neisseria Meningococcal meningitis refers to bacterial meningitis that is brought on by this bacterium. When these microorganisms penetrate into the circulatory system, they may trigger meningococcal meningitis in addition to the typical respiratory tract infections they commonly cause. Teenagers and young adults are the main groups affected by this sickness, which is quite infectious. In residential colleges and military bases, it could start small-scale outbreaks.

A vaccination may aid in illness prevention. Anyone who has come into contact with someone who has meningococcal meningitis, regardless of vaccination status, should take an oral antibiotic in order to ward off the infection.

Monocytogenes Listeria Infection Sausage, fromage and lunchmeats that have not been pasteurized all contain these microorganisms. The most vulnerable groups include expectant women, new parents, seniors, and those with compromised immune systems. Listeria may penetrate the placenta during pregnancy. Infections could cause the infant to pass away in the final stages of pregnancy.

Influenza-causing Haemophilus

The bacterium Haemophilus influenzae B used to be the main contributor to bacterial meningitis in infants. However, the incidence of this particular kind of meningitis has significantly decreased as a result of new vaccines.

What Causes Meningococcal Infection

The two primary causes of meningitis are viruses and bacteria. Meningococcal meningitis is brought on by the bacterium Neisseria meningitidis, which is the most frequent trigger of bacterial meningitis in kids and teenagers. It happens to be the second most typical cause in adults.

The digestive system and the skin are merely a few of the body systems that meningococcal bacteria can infect. The microorganisms may then enter the nervous system through the circulation of blood for unexplained reasons. Meningococcal meningitis is what it creates once it gets there. Additionally, bacteria may reach the neurological system right away following major an operation, head trauma, or an infection.

Risk factors of the Disease

Meningococcal disease risk factors include a number of things, including:

- **Crowded Environments**: Owing to the bacteria's simplicity of spread, staying close to people, especially in camps, dorms, or crowded families, can raise the risk.

- **Trip to Endangered Areas**: There is a higher risk when visiting areas where meningococcal illness is more prevalent.

- **Complement Deficiency**: People who have deficiencies in the immune system's complements are more likely to develop meningococcal illness.

- **Immunodeficiency**: People who have weaker immune systems tend to be more prone to infections, whether as a result of illnesses or treatments like immunosuppressive drugs.

- **Smoking**: Meningococcal illness is more common among smokers, particularly those who frequently smoke a lot.

- **Close contact with infected people**

Staying in close proximity or having intimate contact with an individual who has meningococcal disease, particularly through actions like kissing or sharing utensils, may elevate the risk.

- **Pregnancy**: Women who are pregnant are somewhat more likely to contract meningococcal disease, especially in the third trimester.

The chance of developing severe meningococcal disease is influenced by a number of medical disorders, including sickle cell disease.

Symptoms of Meningococcal Disease

Meningococcal meningitis symptoms can differ from case to case. Signs and symptoms that are more typical include:

- Aching joints
- Severe and lasting headache
- Nausea or diarrhoea
- Comfort with dim lighting
- Neck stiffness
- Sleepiness or trouble waking up
- Unexpected high fever
- Dizziness

- Mental modifications

A very crucial symptom to keep an eye out for is a reddish or purple skin rash, often known as petechiae.

In infants, the following signs will be visible;

- Wailing cry in infants
- Soft area that is tense or enlarged in newborns
- Stiff movements in infants or toddlers
- Irritation
- Rapid respiration
- Laziness
- Persistent sleepiness
- Seizure

Preventive Measures against Meningococcal Infection

Sneezing coughing, kissing, or sharing cigarettes, toothbrushes, or culinary tools are all ways that common viruses and bacteria that cause meningitis might spread.

These actions can aid in meningitis prevention:

- **Maintain proper hygiene**

Never share anything with other people, including toothbrushes, moisturizers for lips, or dining utensils. Additionally, teach children never to give out these items.

- **Hand-washing**

  Washing your hands thoroughly can help stop the transmission of germs. Teach kids to regularly wash their hands, particularly prior to and following using the restroom, being around a lot of people, or stroking animals. Show them the proper technique for washing and rinsing their hands.

- **Keep your health**

  By obtaining enough sleep, exercising frequently, and eating a balanced diet rich in vegetables, whole grains, and cereals, you can keep your immune system strong.

- **Planning your trip**

  If you're going somewhere where meningococcal diseasc is more prevalent, you might want to think about being vaccinated. To reduce exposure, take measures and pay attention to local health recommendations.

- **If you are pregnant**

  If you're expecting a child, watch what you eat. Boiling meat, especially hot dogs and deli meat, to 75 degrees Celsius lowers your chance of contracting listeria. Steer clear of cheeses made from raw milk. Choose cheeses that are made with milk that was pasteurized and are labeled appropriately as such.

Be cautious that you cover your mouth and nose when you sneeze.

- **Educate Others**

  Inform others, as well as yourself, on the symptoms of meningococcal disease. In order to avoid serious consequences, early detection and treatment are often essential.

- **Get Vaccinated**

  In order to stop the spread of meningococcal disease among those in your immediate circle, such as family members or roommates, medical professionals may advise vaccination.

Diagnosis and Medication for Meningococcus Disease

Meningococcal disease can be challenging to diagnose since its symptoms are comparable to those associated with various illnesses, such as the flu. To diagnose this ailment, your doctor has to identify Neisseria meningitidis symptoms in order to collect your blood for testing.

To determine whether the microorganisms can be cultivated (produced), these samples will be delivered to a lab. If the results of the cultures are inconclusive, your doctor may request more tests.

Meningococcal meningitis is a diagnosis that can be supported by tests. The doctor may begin administering antibiotics via an intravenous line, such as ceftriaxone or penicillin. To treat issues brought on by elevated spinal fluid pressure, you or your kid may also require additional medicine. Occasionally, doctors will recommend steroids.

It is crucial to get antibiotics to avoid infection if you or somebody you care about has had close contact with an individual suffering from meningococcal meningitis through saliva or other nasal secretions, for instance at educational institutions, child care, place of employment, or residence.

If you've come into contact with someone who has meningitis, it's equally crucial to consult your doctor. That may be a member of your family, a neighbor, or a coworker. You may require some sort of medicine to prevent getting sick.

Vaccines for Meningococcus Disease

MenACWY vaccines and MenB meningococcal vaccinations are the two vaccine types that are utilized.

All young people from ages 1 - 19 years of age are advised to receive meningococcal vaccinations. Both adults and children receive meningococcal vaccinations in specific circumstances. However, it is advisable to find out from your doctor or that of your child what is ideal for your particular circumstance.

The meningococcal vaccines, including booster injections advisable, are;

Babies

For kids between the ages of two months and ten, the MenACWY vaccine is advisable if they:

- Suffer from a severe immune condition called complement component insufficiency.
- Are a part of an audience that has been discovered as being at increased risk due to a confirmed case of serogroup A, C, W, or Y meningococcal disease.
- Are HIV positive.

- Who travel to or live in countries where serogroup A, C, W, or Y meningococcal disease is prevalent.

Young People

Every 11 to 12-year-old should receive the MenACWY vaccine, followed by a booster dose at age 16. MenB vaccinations are now available for teenagers, ideally between the ages of 16 and 18.

MenB vaccinations are optional for teenagers, although some adolescents and preteens should receive them if they suffer from one of the following conditions:

- Splenic injury
- Have sickle cell disorder
- Belong to a group of people identified as being at higher risk due to an outbreak of MenB illness.

Adults

For older people, the MenACWY immunization is advised if they:

- Suffer from a rare immune condition called complement component insufficiency.
- Have Splenic injury
- Use a complement inhibitor.
- Visit or reside in nations where meningococcal illness of serogroup A, C, W, or Y is prevalent.
- Have sickle cell disorder,

- Have HIV
- Frequently comes into contact with Neisseria meningitidis as a result of their job.
- A military recruit.
- Are a college freshman who lives in a student housing hall who is not up to date on this vaccination.

Why It is Important to get Vaccinated

It's crucial to remember that there are various meningococcal vaccines available that target various bacterial strains. According on aging risk variables, and the incidence of the infection in the area, vaccines are advised. The recommended vaccine regimen must be followed, together with consultation with medical professionals, to provide the best defense against meningococcal illness.

Meningococcal disease vaccination is essential for a number of reasons, including:

- **Lowering the Risk of Spread**

The disease can result in serious and perhaps fatal illnesses such as meningitis, which is a bacteria-related infection of the membranes that cover the brain and spinal cord, and septicemia, which is a bloodstream infection. Getting vaccinated dramatically lowers the risk of contracting these dangerous diseases.

- **Personal Protection**: Those who acquire the vaccine are directly protected as a result of vaccination. It aids their body's defenses in identifying and combating the bacteria. It will protect your kid from infections of the bloodstream in addition to infections of the brain and spinal cord's lining. It also guards against the long-term impairments that are frequently associated with surviving meningococcal illness.

- **Community Protection**: When the majority of people are immunized, the bacteria have less time to spread, safeguarding those individuals who are not immunized. For people who are more susceptible to serious illness, including infants and people with specific medical disorders, this is especially crucial.

- **Safety for Close Contacts**: The total circulation of the bacteria is reduced by decreasing the risk of becoming infected in those who have received the vaccination. Through this, persons who aren't necessarily able to get the vaccine for medical reasons such as allergies or for whom the vaccine might not be as effective such as those with compromised immune systems are indirectly protected.

- **Travel considerations**: Vaccination may be advised or required for admission for travelers, particularly those going to areas where meningococcal illness is more prevalent. This could aid to guarantee your safety when traveling.

Conclusion

Recent advancements in the diagnosis, recovery, and continuous care of patients with the disease have improved the course of meningococcal disease prevention. Meningococcal infection, however, continues to be an important factor of death and disability worldwide despite recent advancements.

Although the release of the serogroup C compounded meningococcal vaccination has been a resounding success, the issue of creating potent vaccines against all illness-causing serogroups for use globally in the fight against the spread of this deadly disease still exists.

To reduce the risk of contracting the disease, it is advised from a health perspective to report to your healthcare provider if you notice any of the listed symptoms.